Dark Psychology

Discover Emotional Manipulation Techniques and Defend Yourself Against Mind Control

Declan Evans

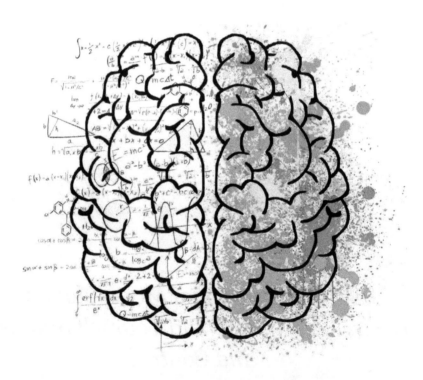

3

Table of Contents

Introduction

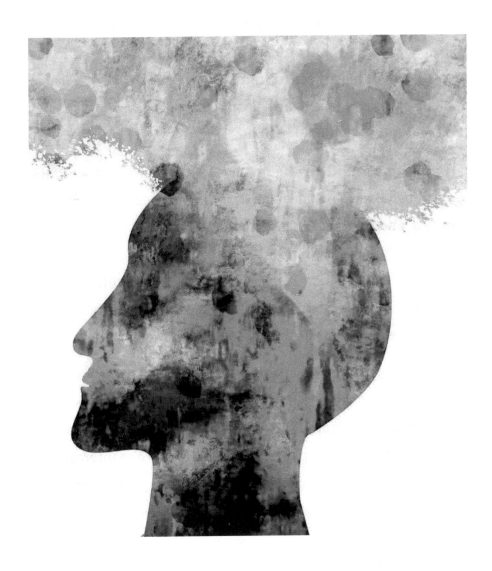

W hat does the term "dark psychology" mean to you? For many, it evokes images of psychopaths, serial killers, and other people who have committed unspeakable acts. Their crimes are so heinous that sometimes it becomes difficult to believe that they have been committed by human beings. These thought processes lead many people to believe that psychology and the dark side go hand in hand.

However, this is far from the reality. Psychology is, after all, the study of behavior. This means that psychology deals with human behavior, and human beings cannot be said to be inherently good or evil. All humans have both the capacity to be good and bad. Psychology simply looks at these behaviors from a different perspective. Psychology can be used for constructive purposes, just as it has been used for destructive purposes.

Understanding the dark side of psychology and coping with sadistic behavior is more important than ever in our violent society. The mind of the serial killer or Hannibal Lecter is just one of many facets that make up human psychology. We're interested as well in what makes a man a hero or a woman touchingly vulnerable. In short, we're interested in the good side as well as the bad side.

Of course, there is some danger in trying to understand the "dark side." It's an easy trap for us to become fascinated by the negative and lose sight of the positive, and vice versa. A few self-styled "experts" on the occult like to convince people that they have been contacted by demons or that they can give them eternal life. They tell their victims that all they must do is give their soul over to their particular brand of belief to achieve their goals.

Unfortunately, there are people who we've come to call prophets of doom. They are obsessed with the pessimistic side of life. Yet, this should not cause us to be afraid of facing the dark side of psychology. However, it is essential to remember that just as many people try to make easy money by preying on the fears of others, so too is a certain amount of skepticism called for when listening to these "experts." The question we have to ask is always, "Is there any hard evidence for their convictions?"

It is important to remember that knowledge is power. It is not something to be feared. The more we know about the dark side, the less harm can be done by those who would take advantage of us. Therefore, we must insist that psychology stays in the realm of science and be open to discoveries to become an increasingly useful tool in our struggle to understand ourselves and our world.

Manipulation and persuasion are two of the most useful strategies in any control-oriented relationship. These skills can make the other person feel good and can even give them an illusion of affection from the controller. The controller may even believe that he or she has some form of respect for their victim. However, it only takes a little knowledge about mind control tactics to recognize their everyday life patterns.

Manipulation is when someone uses or creates an outcome to trigger feelings to get what they want from you. They intend to influence the other person's behavior by emotional means. They may offer love, affection, or even some form of attention. They might promise something that may be appealing to the other person, such as material items or money. Whatever the situation may be, it is something that they hope will cause the other person to act precisely as they want them to.

Persuasion is when someone successfully manipulates another person into doing what they want. This manipulation is done by playing on the other person's emotions and perceptions. It can be done in several ways, including making the other person feel good about themselves, their actions, or their environment. This way of influencing someone usually involves flattery or praise to encourage a positive emotional response.

For the most part, manipulation and persuasion are done unconsciously. This means that when someone is being manipulated or persuaded, they are not fully aware of what is going on. It's essential to recognize these tactics to know when you may be at risk of becoming their victim. Not only do these tactics often lead to problematic situations, but they can also lead to abuse.

Manipulation and persuasion have been linked to several different control-oriented relationships. Fear is one of the most common emotions that we experience, and it can be used as a powerful tool in manipulation and persuasion. Fear affects how we react and how we think about our environment, ourselves, and those around us. The fear itself does not matter as much as the source of it. Fear is a very strong emotion, and it could cause us to make decisions that we usually would not make. It is often triggered by the unknown or by events that we may consider threatening.

Those who would use fear in manipulation and persuasion know this well. They also know how to prey on our feelings of vulnerability to make us feel as if we need them somehow. This could be because of their experience or knowledge in a particular area, ability to offer protection or power over others in the community.

Notes

Chapter 1:
What Is Dark Psychology?

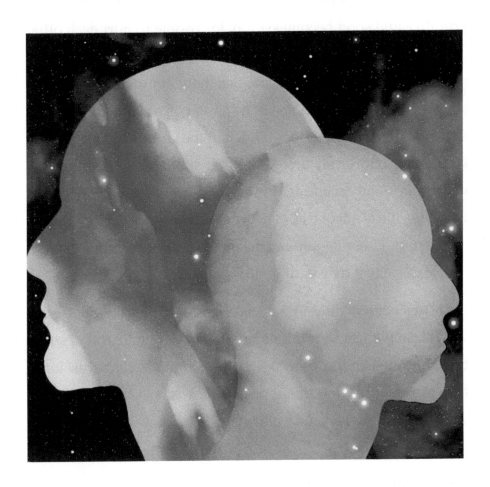

D ark psychology is the study of how to use the dark side—ambiguity, uncertainty, fear, pain, and suffering—to cause massive psychological damage or injury to another person. The use of dark psychology by one human being against another is primitive and soon becomes a way for people to hurt each other daily. These acts are often disguised behind a smile or laugh. Dark psychology does not require complex thought processes. It is usually overt and obvious in its use as a weapon of psychological destruction. It's not a trapdoor hidden in the ground but a cluster of land mines. However, there are often subtle uses of ambiguity, uncertainty, and deception in everyday life that we tend to ignore. In reality, life is full of traps laid by others where if we step wrong, we get hurt. Other people can inevitably cause us serious psychological damage if they wish to do so.

Dark psychology knows no social class or group boundaries. It will take any form to fulfill its mission of psychological destruction. Anyone can use dark psychology, so it's essential to know how to recognize that this type of attack is occurring to protect yourself. The best defense, of course, is to know how and why it works.

The "Dark" in Dark Psychology

The light represents good intentions in relationships. The dark represents negative intentions in relationships. For psychological purposes, life is divided into those that have the light of goodness in their hearts, actions, and minds; and those touched by darkness of some sort. Those with the ability to influence people for good or bad are often referred to as "dark wizards." If one is touched by darkness, it means they can hurt another person psychologically for their purposes. Evil exists in human relationships, and dark psychology is designed to use this evil to harm another person through nonverbal communication.

The study of dark psychology has been part of the human condition since the beginning of time, but formal study to use this knowledge for good purposes has yet to take form. The psychologist Carl Jung was once quoted as saying, "Everything that irritates us about others can lead us to an understanding of ourselves." This is a truism for the field of dark psychology, which delves into the darker side of human relationships and communication. However, there is a way to gain insight from these interactions if viewed within a framework for positive personal growth and change.

Dark psychology should be studied to understand how it works, then used, when needed, to prevent psychopaths from harming others and themselves. Knowledge of dark psychology can be used to help others but also to protect ourselves from the acts of others.

Why Bother with Dark Psychology?

Life is a study of human relationships and communication. Every relationship has its dark side that can be used against us if we don't know how and why it works, or worse—if we don't even know it exists. The worst problems in life occur between people who have no idea how their words and actions affect others or themselves. The challenge facing all of us daily is to learn how to understand and control our own emotions. This alone is the most important lesson we need to know. Dark psychology simply makes this task more interesting and enlightening. Dark psychology is the study of relationships between human beings who have a dark side that they use with great skill against others. Understanding dark psychology can be very useful, especially when dealing with those who have no moral or social compass to guide them in their thoughts or actions.

While cruel and evil people exist, they are often not psychopaths or sociopaths. The majority of those who harm others daily do so because they want to feel great about themselves, not just because they follow some deep-rooted psychological or are emotionally dysfunctional. In fact, these people usually have many friends and family who like them. They simply use dark psychology as a tool for manipulation without realizing it.

The Power of Dark Psychology

People who are skilled at using the dark side in their relationships with others have a natural advantage. It may not be clear at first, but this advantage can be extremely helpful in achieving goals and objectives. The beauty of the dark side is that it is unconscious most of the time and can be used without worrying about it to achieve positive ends.

Let's face it, life on earth is often mundane and boring. The use of dark psychology helps provide interest and excitement to otherwise dull lives. If you can use it to help others as well, then it can be a powerful tool. The best way to use it is to be aware of its existence and how it works and then decide what you will do with the information when needed. In addition to being a powerful tool for manipulation, dark psychology can be used to enhance our own lives. These people usually have higher self-esteem, more friends, better jobs, and are generally more successful in life. They may not be happy people on the whole, but they certainly are effective and frequently achieve their goals.

Dark Psychology in the World

Dark psychology studies man's less desirable traits along with their social and economic implications. Dark Psychology includes such issues as violence, aggression, bullying, lying, greed, selfishness, and indifference. Although people are involved with dark psychology in the world, it can be studied in animals, too.

As of yet, we cannot reliably predict when a person will respond with dark psychology. We cannot determine which events or situations will set someone off into a violent rage, and we cannot say what might trigger an act of bullying.

The field is multidisciplinary, which means it takes ideas from biology, economics, cognitive science, and many other branches of science. Dark Psychology prepares students for careers with applied use, including law enforcement, research, social services, and more. The area is also in its early stages, and the terminology may change, but for now, it is a new branch of psychology.

Anything that affects our lives can be good or bad, and Dark Psychology includes both. When you think of Dark Psychology, you may think of violent or greedy people. But, many positive things have come from studying the dark side of human nature, such as helping us understand the reasons why we may behave in a certain way, a way that is not considered to be socially acceptable.

Notes

Chapter 2:
Techniques of Dark Psychology

The techniques of dark psychology encompass the methods of persuasion and influence people use with morally dubious motivations. The intent of such persuasion is often to alter the perception and behavior of their victims towards something they consider desirable. These may be actions that would be illegal or unethical when carried out by conventional means or actions that are considered acceptable but are carried out in a way that is significantly more powerful than necessary in order to exert power over a victim. Techniques such as guilt manipulation, lying, and slander form part of this set of tools.

Manipulation

The truth is that we all manipulate one another, consciously or unconsciously. Whether it be getting a partner to do what we want or trying to sell a product or idea, manipulation is part of life

It is a common myth that manipulation is in itself immoral or unethical. The successful salesman, for example, relies on his ability to manipulate customers in order to get them to buy his product. Yet we admire the salesmanship of the good salesman. We understand that he cannot make a sale unless he can get his customer to buy something, and we accept this fact as a part of life in our consumer society.

The only time manipulation becomes evil is when it becomes abusive or coercive. For example, if a boyfriend threatens his girlfriend with harm unless she has sex with him, he is using an evil form of manipulation.

The same is true with salesmen or women whose job it is to coerce us into doing things we might not otherwise do. Take a car salesperson, for example. He needs to use manipulation tactics to get you to buy the car he is trying to sell you. But at the same time, he cannot be completely honest with you because that would put him out of business! Every customer who comes into his showroom has already decided they are going to buy a car. It's all a matter of when and how much it will cost them. The salesman is just a part of the process each customer must go through in their minds to arrive at a decision.

The true art of manipulation is understanding the inner workings of your victim's mind and finding ways to influence them without making them feel manipulated. It requires a degree of self-knowledge, insight, and feeling sympathy for the person you are manipulating. If you can accomplish that feat, you have mastered one of the most powerful life skills.

Some tips to help you learn the art of manipulation.

Know your victim

To be a good manipulator, you need to know your victim intimately. Get to know their likes and dislikes, personality quirks, hopes and fears, and their dreams and ambitions. You should find out what they want more than anything else in the world. That is the key to manipulating them!

Do not simply ask them what they want, though. Instead, watch their behavior with a keen eye and observe what they do when they reach out for something they want.

Next, start the process of learning their weaknesses. Everyone has them. Even you! It's a good idea to analyze your own weak points, so you know what to avoid in your victims' minds when it comes time to manipulate them.

Finally, learn their personality type. People tend to belong to one of the 4 basic personality types: extrovert, introvert, thinker, or feeler. Knowing your victim's personality type will help you understand how to manipulate them into doing what you want.

Know yourself

To be a good manipulator, you need to know yourself as well. For example, do you tend to be more extroverted or introverted? If you are an extrovert, it is easier for you to manipulate those around you because they tend to cooperate with extroverts who share their energy and enthusiasm. If you are introverted, you tend to be more private and less likely to share your mind with others. As a result, others will not be as willing to give you what you want when they get tired of listening to your demands.

You also need to keep track of your weak points so that when the time comes, you dodge an attack on those weaknesses by your victims.

Know the situation

There are many ways to manipulate someone into doing something they would not normally do otherwise. You need to understand how each method of manipulation will affect your victim. The best approach for you depends on what you are trying to accomplish and how you want the results of your manipulation to appear.

Do not forget that desires easily manipulate people. Their self-interest is a powerful weapon in the hands of a good manipulator.

Persuasion

Lasting change can happen in many ways, but it all begins with persuasive communication. There are three main types of persuasion: rational, informational, and emotional. We all use these techniques when we want to get someone to do what we want them to do.

Good persuasive writing uses all three forms of persuasion to be effective. Use as much information as possible without overdoing it. Use rhetorical devices wisely to get your point across in the most persuasive manner possible while at the same time maintaining credibility.

Think about what you are trying to say, and then select the best combination of techniques to communicate your message effectively. It is needed a great deal of trial and error. You might have to write something a dozen times before you get it right. Persuasion is always an art!

Informational Persuasion

This form of persuasion is used when the main goal of the communication is to inform someone about something they didn't recognize from the past or difficult for them to understand on their own.

Persuasion happens when you present the information in a way that causes the other person to learn, experience, or discover something on their own. It is not just giving someone a lecture; it is guiding them through an experience.

Learning by doing can be very powerful because it makes the information more real to them than merely reading a book about it. It also makes your message stick with them longer and be more likely to change their behavior.

Here are some examples of informational persuasion:

Self-Directed Learning

This form of persuasion is used when the communication goal is to teach someone something they will be able to use to successfully perform a task.

Seldom will anyone learn anything by just being told how to do it. They have to figure it out on their own, or they will never really understand it. Even small children require this kind of learning in order for them to truly understand something. The most successful way for children to learn is by doing it on their own.

We learn and change our behavior when we are actively involved in the learning process. Nothing beats the hands-on approach.

Example of Self-Directed Learning:

A book on "How to make a good presentation" is a highly informative topic, but it does not lend itself to an effective persuasive technique because it is hard to do yourself, and there will be no one around to see how well you do. You are just reading a book.

Self-directed learning is much more effective.

"How to make a good presentation in front of your class" is a much better topic for self-directed learning because you can learn how to make a good presentation in front of your class, and then you can show the world how well you learned it.

This form of persuasion requires that the person being persuaded go through an experience to understand it, making it stick with them longer and be more likely to change their behavior.

Playing to Emotions (Emotional Persuasion)

Emotional appeals are extremely powerful. They change behavior and motivate people to act. People often do things to either gain approval or avoid disapproval. When you can make someone lose face or feel embarrassed, you can influence their behavior a lot easier than someone who does not have that power over them.

When you want someone to feel something strongly and then do something due to that feeling, it is very powerful indeed.

Example of Playing to Emotions:

"There are starving children in Africa, and it is your fault because you have not donated any money. By donating just two dollars a day, you can save a child's life!"

This kind of play on emotion is very effective because the person being persuaded feels guilt over letting a child die, so they donate the money.

Another example of playing to emotions is to appeal to the person's ego. You want to make them feel important or powerful. Sometimes you can appeal to both their pride and their guilt simultaneously, which makes for a powerful combination.

Types of persuasion

Moral licensing has been proven to play a substantial role in the use of morally dubious persuasion tactics. When people commit an act that is considered good or ethical, they automatically feel licensed to carry out unrelated devious, unethical actions in the future. This is particularly true when they are under the influence of alcohol and narcotics, as they then feel less guilt. Once a person has done something conscionably wrong, they feel more comfortable doing something similar in the future. This is because they look at themselves as a person who carries out both good and bad deeds. This is a justification that they use to overcome their guilt.

An attitude of mind that favors persuasion tactics is considered morally dubious, such as lying. It's not enough for the individual to break moral rules. They must also possess the belief that certain acts are, in fact, morally justified. There are many different types of people who are more likely to possess a self-serving attitude – for example, individuals chosen for leadership positions. People who got high scores on the Narcissistic Personality Inventory also show signs of having a self-serving attitude, as they believe that, in general, the world is full of injustices based on those less worthy than them. Another factor influencing an individual's attitude is whether they come from a family in which deceitful acts were accepted and common.

High self-esteem can lead to the use of persuasion tactics that are considered morally dubious. This is because a person with high self-esteem finds it easier to control their guilty feelings. A low level of self-esteem can have the opposite effect and makes people more likely to feel more guilt, making them less likely to carry out unethical acts. People who have a low level of self-esteem are also less likely to use persuasion tactics that are considered morally dubious.

Being able to be completely separate from the consequences of our actions can lead to the use of persuasion tactics considered morally dubious by many. A person capable of this can temporarily remove themselves emotionally from the act, making it easier for them to do whatever they like. The use of persuasion tactics that are considered morally dubious may become a lifestyle, as morals or feelings do not hold them back.

Notes

Chapter 3:
Dark Psychology Traits

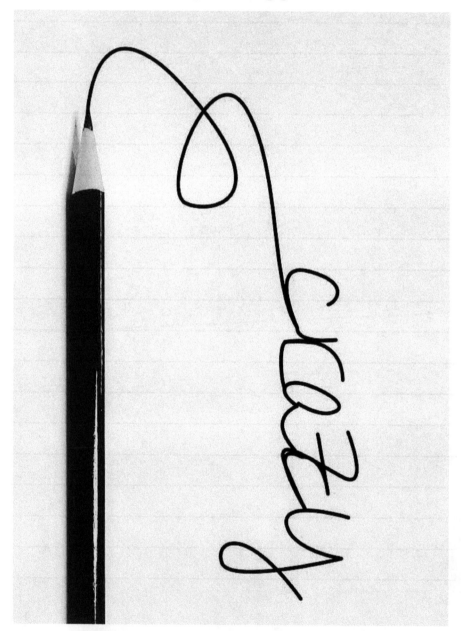

What is Narcissism?

T he term narcissism is from the name of the Greek mythological character Narcissus. It refers to those who exhibit traits of excessive self-love and lack of self-awareness. While all ordinary people have some degree of narcissism, people with Narcissistic Personality Disorder are so excessively narcissistic that they use others to feed their own needs and desires. A narcissistic person lacks empathy and is highly exploitative; he takes what he wants without caring about the consequences for others or even for himself in the long term. He is an automaton, incapable of making emotional connections and incapable of caring about others.

The narcissist has an incredible sense of entitlement and expects to be treated as special.

Narcissists frequently have other personality disorders, such as borderline, histrionic, or anti-social personality disorder. They are also likely to be substance abusers or addicts; they need their substance(s) to fuel their fragile false self and the image of their grandiosity projected to the world.

Narcissists are also frequently paranoid, which means that they are hypersensitive to any perceived threat. They tend to read hidden meanings into innocent remarks or gestures.

As a result of their extremely fragile self-esteem (more often than not, completely unfounded), narcissists feel the need to protect themselves from the slightest insult or disagreement and react with rage and hostility to any slight criticism or disagreement; they cannot handle being ignored, overlooked, or slighted in any way. They consider conflict to be a form of attack. Narcissists are prone to fits of intense rage and anger when threatened.

The narcissist is convinced that he is superior, more important, more intelligent than others, and entitled to special treatment. He considers himself uniquely talented and often has an exaggerated sense of achievements and abilities. He may also tend toward exaggeration or lying on his resume, in his accomplishments or skills, to make himself look better than he is. Narcissists are often highly critical of others and enjoy seeing other people caught in their web of lies and deceptions.

The narcissist is a master manipulator who is often charming yet ruthless. He knows how to 'talk' his way into all kinds of situations, especially by making himself look good or by making you feel sorry for him. He knows how to 'play' people like a puppet master to get them to do what he wants.

What is Machiavellianism

The term Machiavellianism is derived from the name of the Italian Renaissance diplomat and writer Niccolò di Bernardo dei Machiavelli. The term refers to those who are manipulative, scheming, self-serving and, opportunistic. They are highly intelligent but use their intelligence to manipulate others for their own benefit. They use lies, deceit, and manipulation to get their way.

They are extremely unflappable and never show any sign of weakness.

Machiavellians tend toward callousness, lack of empathy, and the inability to feel remorse or guilt even when confronted with evidence that their behavior was harmful to others. They tend to be cynical and believe that the end justifies the means.

What is a Psychopath?

The term is derived from the Greek words *psykhe* and *pathos,* meaning brain and suffering, respectively (meaning suffering of the mind). It refers to an individual with an antisocial personality disorder (ASPD). In everyday language, the psychopath can refer to any criminal or deviant person. Contrary to popular misconceptions, not all psychopaths are killers, and most of them live outside prisons. Many of them are successful in the business world as entrepreneurs, corporate leaders, and politicians.

Psychopaths have a callous disregard for the feelings of others, including their family and friends. They use people for their gain without any regard for them as humans. Psychopaths are highly manipulative and only see others as objects or targets in their manipulation games. They learn to mimic emotions, but they don't experience emotions like normal people do.

What is Sadism?

Sadists derive pleasure from inflicting pain and humiliating others. They enjoy seeing their victims suffer and get off on not only hurting others but ruining their lives as well.

The sadist is a master at reading people and knows just how to push their buttons to inflict the most pain without arousing suspicion. The more pain and humiliation he can inflict, the better; he gets off on it. The sadist is also a hypocrite; he considers himself a moral person, but his behavior is the exact opposite of what he preaches.

The sadist is arrogant and highly opinionated, unaware of the hypocrisy of his own beliefs, and often intolerant to other opinions. He considers himself superior to others and always has to be in control. He is competitive with others and spiteful when he loses. The sadist enjoys manipulating others and playing human torture games; he derives pleasure from making people suffer for his own enjoyment. The sadist often comes from a troubled background and has suffered abuse and neglect in his formative years. He was often bullied, humiliated, beaten, and rejected by others in his childhood. He felt powerless and helpless during his youth; he learned that the only way to gain the upper hand was through violence and aggression. As a result, he developed an overwhelming need to control his environment; he became sadistic as a way to feel better about himself.

Notes

Chapter 4:
Manipulation in Dark Psychology

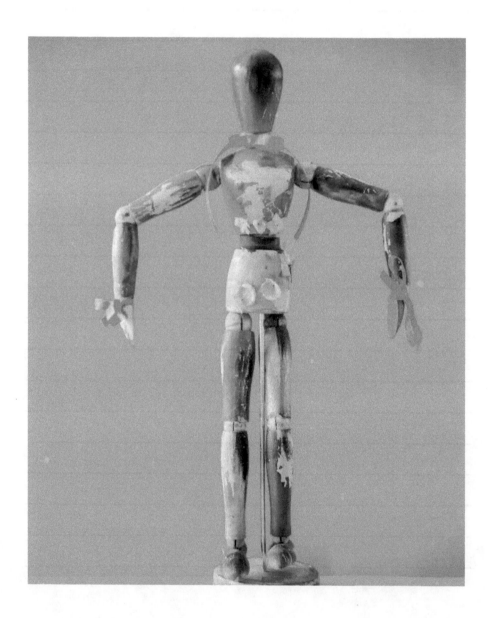

M an is a social animal where his survival and progress depend largely on his ability to influence other people. Manipulation is the process of guiding and controlling the behavior of others through specific methods. It is a process that can be used for both good and bad purposes.

Manipulation is a tool that we employ to achieve our own goals. However, its usefulness should not blind us to its inherent dangers. The negative consequences of manipulation far outweigh the positive ones. To avoid this, we must first understand the concept thoroughly and realize when it's being used against our loved ones or us.

History of Manipulation

Manipulation has been practiced ever since the beginning of man. Manipulation was used in ancient times for achieving goals. In ancient warfare, there was an art of war designed to fool and outsmart your enemy. The art of psychological warfare has been around for a long time.

In ancient times, manipulators used to trick their enemy in every possible way. They used to misguide them about their objectives and intentions. They used to deceive them to win the warfare. In the same way, business people and politicians use psychological manipulation to achieve their goals. Manipulation is employed by everyone in some or another.

Manipulation in Business

The definition mentioned above of manipulation can be applied to business also. The businessmen apply these methods on a large scale for increasing their sales. Salesmen use psychological methods to enhance their sales. They mislead the customers about the quality and usefulness of a product and convince them by making false claims about their product. Sometimes, they even lie to the customers about the product features in order to make a sale. Similarly, politicians also use psychological manipulation to promote their political careers.

Manipulation within Family

The same methods of manipulation are employed by people within a family as well. In some cases, husband or wife employs these methods for getting what they want from each other. Sometimes parents use these methods to fulfill their selfish desires from their children and vice versa.

Manipulation in Politics

In politics, this art is used by politicians to achieve success. Politicians mislead people by misrepresenting facts and figures. They often lie about their achievements and programs to gain people's trust to be elected as a political representative of a nation.

Manipulation within Religion

In religion, manipulation is being used by religious leaders to promote their own beliefs. They also misguide the people by misrepresenting facts and figures. They lie to the people about the nature of their religious beliefs. These acts are not justified at all, but they are still being employed to achieve their selfish desires.

Manipulation in Society

In society, these methods are used by everyone in some way or other for achieving their personal goals and agenda. People often employ these methods for fulfilling their needs and wishes without taking others into consideration.

How to Detect and Avoid Manipulation

The easiest way to detect manipulation is to remain mindful of your emotions. When you feel angry, upset, frustrated, or hurt, stop and think about how you arrived at that feeling state.

Manipulation attempts are often obvious when you're conscious of what to look for. Manipulators often use such methods as shaming, guilt, sex, threats, and violence to get what they want.

If you find yourself questioning the motives of the manipulator, they are probably doing it intentionally.

Manipulation is often an art form that's subtle and complex.

It's a good idea to read up on manipulation, ways to spot it, and how to avoid being manipulated yourself. Knowledge is power when it comes to manipulation. It's also important to remember that manipulation should not be confused with influence or persuasion. Once you understand the difference between manipulation and influence, you'll be in a better position to know when someone is manipulating you.

Manipulation can be a difficult issue to deal with. It's best to avoid it altogether by maintaining healthy relationships in your life where manipulation isn't present.

While it can be an uncomfortable feeling, remember that you don't have to put up with being manipulated.

Acknowledge the fact that you're being manipulated and take steps to change the situation.

Learning to tell the difference between healthy relationships and manipulative ones can help put you in a better position to avoid manipulation.

Trust your instincts. If something doesn't feel right, it probably isn't.

Take care of your life by making decisions that are best for you, regardless of what others will think of you or what they want you to do.

If a situation makes you uncomfortable, get out of it as quickly as possible. Nothing good can come from putting yourself in an uncomfortable situation that could potentially be harmful to you somehow. If you've been manipulated into believing something untrue, get the facts and correct the misunderstanding as quickly as possible.

Reject being an unwilling participant in other people's plans. Know your limits and know when to say no.

It can be difficult to avoid manipulation entirely with all of the dishonest characters out there. It's usually better to talk about your problems than just going along with what everyone else is doing just to fit in or avoid being criticized for questioning what others believe or are doing.

Notes

Chapter 5:
How to Use Manipulation

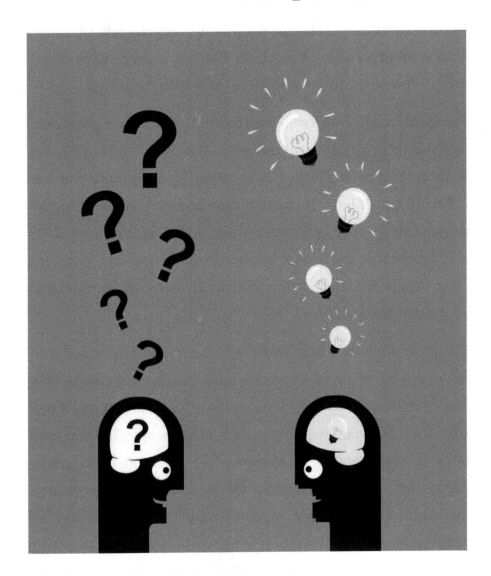

S ome people become victims of manipulation, but others use manipulation for achieving their goals. For those people who are using manipulation, it is the best way to gain what they want from others. It is a common fact that humans have always used different strategies to achieve success in their lives.

Manipulation can work well as a tool for the success of people and help fulfill their needs and interests. Manipulation is defined as the act of controlling or fooling someone by using one's power to influence him or her. This activity may be done consciously or unconsciously by causing certain feelings in the opposite party. Usually, people who are good at manipulation are experts in moving other people, and they have a high ability to handle various situations that occur daily.

Manipulation is used in different ways and for different purposes. There is a positive and a negative purpose. There are some basic strategies that are used during manipulation. The first one is persuasion. It is a good way to persuade other people, but you must be careful when you use this strategy because it can damage both parties if it is not done correctly. The second one is called disarming, and it is used to disarm another person to make them feel comfortable with the situation so they will agree with your plan or idea. This method will work well when you know how to make people feel comfortable with you and your personality.

Manipulation happens in many situations, but most people use it to get what they want from other people. They use their power to influence other people, so they will agree with their plan or idea. If you are planning to use manipulation for achieving success, you must be skilled enough and must have the ability to control the situation because your success depends on your performance.

We can find it in our personal or professional lives. Knowing the facts that manipulation has both positive and negative effects on people, it is important to be careful when using it.

In order to use this strategy successfully, you must be skilled enough and know the factors that make people trust you. You must be honest and sincere with your words and have a positive approach because the success of your career is in your own hands.

You need to know when to use this strategy and when not to use it. You should never use manipulation as a way of living because you will not succeed in the end. You must make sure that you are using strategies that will help you gain a good reputation and success in your life because if you aren't using them for a useful purpose, they may cost you much more than you think in the future. When you are using manipulation, you must make sure that you are not hurting other people to achieve your goals.

It is good to know how this strategy can be used for achieving success, but it will harm you if you use it for personal gains and purposes.

When people are using manipulation, they must have the ability to control other people and must know when to use this strategy. In order to use the manipulation effectively, you must have a positive approach and honesty in your words because the effect of this strategy will depend on your performance in the end. There are also some questions that you must ask yourself before using manipulation. The first one is: " Do I need to use this or not? How far do I want to go with this strategy? "

One of the most popular strategies for gaining success is manipulation. It can be used for different needs and purposes, but mostly it is used for deceiving people and for good behavior.

This strategy can be used in many situations. If you are planning to use manipulation for achieving success, you must be skilled enough. You must have the ability to control the situation to have a positive outcome.

There are some factors that you must take into consideration before using manipulation. This strategy can backfire on you if you are not using it properly.

Manipulation in the World Today

Manipulation in the world today is commonplace. It is everywhere. There is nowhere you can go without feeling or seeing it. When we think about manipulation, we tend to think of ways to get what we want out of someone. That seems to be one straightforward way of manipulating someone into doing something or saying something they may not have done if they had been given a choice.

In our world today, it is probably the most common form of manipulation. When dealing with salespeople and the endless stream of advertisements, we are bombarded with every day in almost every aspect of our lives. We are being manipulated to buy, buy and buy again. Manipulation tactics such as "Limited Time Only," "For a Limited Time Only," or "For a Very Limited Time" are used to entice us into buying a product that we felt may have been out of reach financially. This is a form of manipulation on the customer that will eventually lead them into buying that product. The "Limited Time Only" tactic is used in advertising all the time to draw people into their products and services. For example, "Hurry Hurry," "Act Now," or my favorite one is "Limited Quantity." Notice how your attention is being drawn to it.

Another example is the salesperson who will act in a very conversational tone of voice as if they are on our side and supporting us all the way. When they talk to us, we can feel their excitement about what they are selling and want a part of it. We want to be excited about what they are selling, but most importantly, we want them to be excited about their selling. We do not realize that they are manipulating us into feeling this way, but on the other hand, it is nothing out of the ordinary as they have been doing this to everyone else all day long. We are probably not the only customers they have talked to today, and we will not be the last either.

When it comes to advertising, manipulation tactics create an image or a feeling about a product or service. For example, when we see an ad for a luxury car and the background is a beautiful beach with clear blue waters. In the foreground is a very expensive-looking car. The message being conveyed to us is that if you buy this car, you will be able to enjoy the same lifestyle as those on the beach. A manipulation tactic used in advertising (which appears on TV) is to create an image or desire for something by using celebrities in their ads. They are using the fact that we would like to be like them, either for their looks or lifestyle. It is a form of manipulation to get us (the public) to buy the product they are promoting. Also, to manipulate is to control; when you see an ad with a celebrity in it, the message being given to you is that if you buy this product, it will make you look like (or have) the lifestyle of that celebrity.

Another type of manipulation is when someone wants something so much but does not have enough money to pay for it, so they get a loan. The loan gives us what we want, but at the same time, we have now gone into debt and will have to pay it off in the future. The thing we want becomes a necessity, and we have to get it.

In our world today, manipulation is everywhere and everything around us. When people want you to do something or tell you something just because they want you to know it, they are manipulative. The whole world is being controlled by this way of thinking and acting to obtain the most money for themselves at all costs as fast as they can get it.

Manipulation in our world today is used in almost any aspect you can think of. If you ask a person about something on the street for the time, they will say, "What's it to ya?" When you do not answer their question, they will repeatedly ask until they get an answer from you. Or when you say something to someone or even correct them, they will hear what you are saying, but inwardly, they think it is not true. They are thinking that there is no way you know what you are talking about when what is happening is they do not want to accept the truth of what you are saying, or they feel that you are trying to make them look stupid. This also shows how we can be manipulated in our everyday lives.

In this world today, we cannot get away from manipulation, whether we like it or not, as it has become normal for us to deal with it every day of our lives in some way. We are manipulated in the simplest way through advertising and sales pitches. We are manipulated to eat what we have never even thought about before. Even our banks and financial institutions manipulate us through our bank statements as they make it appear as if you owe them money when you do not.

Manipulation is everywhere today that it almost seems as if there is no escape from it. As mentioned earlier, it is a way of thinking and acting to get what they want. Whatever it is they want, whatever it takes to get it, that is how they will do it. They believe in getting their way instead of negotiating a solution that both parties are happy with. It is almost as if their attitude towards life and the needs of others do not matter. Everything is all about them and their needs. Manipulation is used in advertising today to create a feeling or an image about a certain product, which will be reflected by the public who will buy them. Also, manipulation is used when celebrities are used in our advertising because we would like to be like them (to have their lifestyles) or become who they are.

Manipulation is present everywhere today, irrespective of the type of society that you live in; it is indeed a part of our world that has significantly evolved throughout time. Manipulation is so extreme nowadays that we do not even realize how badly we are being manipulated. It is an everyday thing for us, and it has become a normal thing for us to deal with. We must think about this carefully in order to make a change and start thinking about others when we are using or being manipulated by others.

Notes

Chapter 6:
Psychological Manipulation Techniques?

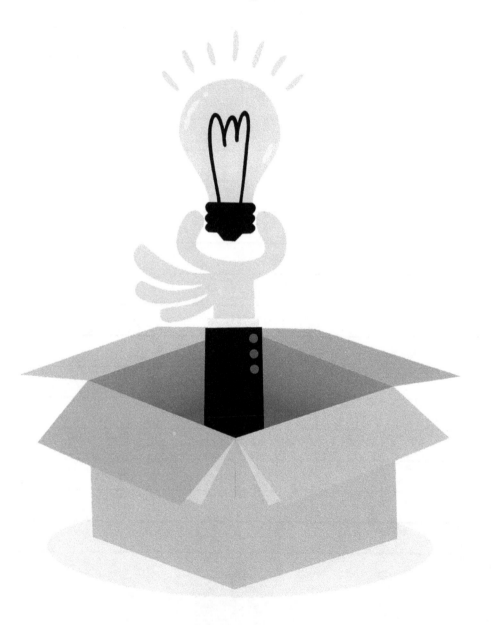

I t is quite easy to get people to do what you want them to do without their knowing it. Psychological manipulation is an art used by powerful people in every sector of society. This form of manipulation has been practiced for centuries and is still used in present times.

These are the most common techniques employed in psychological manipulation. These will be used to manipulate other people when you want to get your way.

1. Aggressive and Passive-Aggressive Manipulation

Many people, when they want to achieve something, use aggressive manipulation while some others would use passive-aggressive manipulation. Both are alike in a way, but there are differences between them too.

2. Bait and Switch

This is a technique used to get people to do the thing you want them to do. You will first attract people with an attractive bait, and once they are interested, you will switch the bait with something else. This is an effective technique used in marketing many products.

3. Bipolar Manipulation

This method aims at reversing the negativity of a situation so that the manipulator can get what he wants from his victim. First, the manipulator will act in a way that will make his victim think he is his enemy, and then when his victim feels safe, he will start acting friendly with him. This way the manipulator can control his victim's actions more easily.

4. Bullying

The people who use this method of manipulation are usually bullies when they want something from someone else. They would use verbal insults to pressure their victims into doing what they want. Some bullies tend to use physical force to intimidate their victims.

5. Covert Hypnosis

This is a type of manipulation that is usually done through suggestion or using hypnosis to influence other people. People who use this method have learned how to hypnotize people without using hypnosis.

6. Deliberate Deception

The manipulator will lie to his victim about what he wants from him, use false promises and make fake guarantees. He will also persuade and manipulate his victim into believing that he is a genuine person who needs their help. These lies are intended to give the victim a sense of security that he can trust and believe in his sincerity. He will always act as if the victim is in control of their relationship and make it seem as if he only wants the best for them. This is something that professional con artists are very good at; they know how to manipulate their victims into believing everything they say or do is for the victim's own good, although they are doing the complete opposite.

7. Demonization

This is one of the best methods used in manipulating other people. This method is often used by politicians to persuade people to go against their enemies and vote for them in an election. The manipulator will convince his victim that the other person is evil and should be killed or shouldn't be associated with.

8. Denial

Most people are aware of this manipulation technique. When something bad happens, and the person wants to get out of it by making the other person believe it was not their fault, they tend to use denial. If you have done something you are not supposed to do, you should avoid using this technique, or you would just end up creating more problems for yourself.

9. Guilt Manipulation

People who employ this technique make their victims feel guilty. They use this technique to make their victims do things they want. This is one of the most powerful methods used in manipulation since people usually do what they can to avoid feeling guilty. Nowadays, some people would use the media to make people feel so guilty about the bad habits that they would not be able to sleep at night because of guilt, and some would even commit suicide because of it.

10. Hypnotic Persuasion

This is used by hypnotists. This method is prevalent among religious leaders who use it to make their congregation do what they want. But, this is not a technique for the weak.

When someone is being hypnotized, they will be very focused on what the hypnotist is saying and doing. They will stare at the hypnotist's eyes with their own eyes wide open in complete fascination.

11. Lying

Lying is one way the manipulator can use to achieve what he wants from you. Lying is an effective way of manipulation since most people would rather believe a lie than the truth. An indirect manipulation is an underhanded way of manipulation, such as telling white lies and lies by omission. Direct manipulation is a blatantly obvious approach to manipulate the other person, such as shouting and yelling out blatant lies.

It would be easy for you to spot a liar if they are direct because they will most likely be making more facial movements. When someone tells a lie, their voice might change or tense up in different ways, providing clues.

12. Pressuring

This method will be employed by people who want to force their victims to do what they want them to do. They would use some form of pressure such as threat or intimidation so that their victims will give in and do what they want.

Notes

Chapter 7:
Mind Control

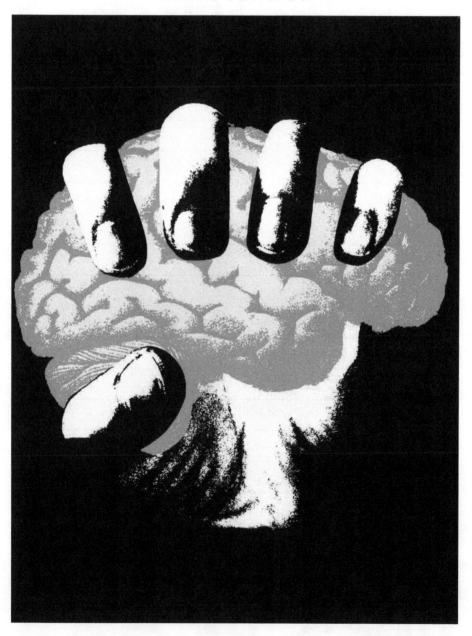

M ind control (also known as Behavior Modification) is a set of techniques designed to influence a human being's behavior, or other organisms, without the use of drugs (which tend to have side-effects), pain, or coercion. Techniques intended to bring about permanent behavioral change, usually called "mind control," are typically called "brainwashing" if done in a coercive programmatic way; the term brainwashing is also used if done by high-pressure sales tactics. "Psychological manipulation" may be used to refer to softer forms of persuasion (e.g., jiu-jitsu).

The goal of mind control is often surreptitious manipulation—to change the way people perceive reality, how they behave, and what information they are capable of processing. For example, a government might attempt to control citizens' behavior so that they can be influenced in how they vote by using propaganda and "information warfare."

Methods and effects

There are four main methods used to achieve mind control:

Information control

Information control is achieved by limiting access to information outside the control of the organization. This is used by groups such as cults that will isolate their members from all current and/or former affiliations, thus requiring them to depend exclusively on the group's beliefs and teachings.

Financial control

Financial control involves limiting a target's access to funds and material goods. This creates a dependency on the organization or leader and is often used in cults that provide food, shelter, etc., and require donations.

Performance control

Performance control is achieved by monitoring and regulating the actions of the target. This can be achieved by requiring the target to get approval for everything they do and making them ask permission to carry out any task or action.

Psychological control

Psychological control works by manipulating the thoughts, feelings, and actions of individuals through various techniques. This can be achieved by using multiple pressures and influences brought to bear on the individual, including peer-pressure, emotional stress, intimidation, threats, behavior modification techniques, and hypnosis.

Some of these techniques are shown to be effective at an amazingly early age in some individuals (infant programming). Techniques such as brainwashing or mind control do not always include violence. Government agencies in the United States have reportedly used hypnosis for interrogation purposes in attempts to get suspects to reveal information that they would not otherwise reveal.

Behavioral control is control by punishment and reward. The use of punishment to control behavior is called "aversive control." Governments or social systems' operant conditioning techniques to induce specific behaviors are called "operant conditioning." Operant conditioning and aversive control are not always distinct, but in some cases, behavior modification and coercive persuasion can be distinguished. Punishment is often simply referred to as "negative" reinforcement when the goal is to eliminate the undesirable behavior, and positive reinforcement when the goal is to strengthen an already desired behavior.

Reward can be classified as either positive or negative. Positive reinforcement occurs when a behavior is followed by a pleasurable stimulus to the individual, so the person continues the action. Negative reinforcement occurs when a behavior leads to removing an unpleasant stimulus, and the behavior will increase. Punishment can also be classified as either positive or negative. Positive punishment occurs when a behavior is followed by an aversive stimulus, and the unwanted behavior decreases.

Non-physical techniques can be broken down into two main categories: those that require the cooperation of the subject and those that do not. The latter is far more effective, as they can usually be used against "non-cooperative" subjects.

A Deep Dive into Mind Control

Consciousness is a fragile, elusive phenomenon. The mind is also a delicate and complex organ that humans often take for granted. Yet, in reality, humans are only about 60 or 70% proactive in their daily lives around the globe. Many people are controlled by external factors and events - rather than being the masters of their own destiny. Mind control has been used for centuries to manipulate human behavior and keep vast populations under control.

This dark topic has been shrouded in mystery for years, but research and media coverage of mind control has emerged from obscurity in recent times. The concept is simple enough: brainwash or control individuals' minds to manipulate their decisions, perceptions, and behaviors.

This idea used to be a popular concept in science fiction stories; many movies explored the ramifications of mind control and brainwashing experiments on unsuspecting human subjects. However, these days it is becoming an ever-increasing reality in our everyday lives.

Consciousness, Cognition, and Behavior

To understand brainwashing techniques and mind control strategies, it's crucial to have a basic understanding of cognition and behavior. This includes the use of these tactics and their adverse impacts on individuals subjected to them.

The Biology of Behavior

A human brain is a biological machine that we've yet to understand fully. The brain is divided into three main parts: the hindbrain, midbrain, and forebrain. They are responsible for processing data from the environment, regulating your body's systems and emotions, and interpreting information from your five senses. The latter of these is where communication between your mind and the world outside begins to take shape.

Brain Mechanisms that Shape Behavior

The mind is the interface between you and your environment. It is your conscious experience of the world around you and a repository for all your memories, ideas, and beliefs. Your perception of the world largely shapes your behavior. This is why it's important to understand how cognition works to see how mind control tactics and strategies work in action.

Behavior modification is constantly occurring in our everyday lives. People are influenced by friends, family, peers, and the media. Your brain automatically rewards you with a pleasurable response when you do something appropriate or support your goals. Conversely, you experience negative responses from your brain when you perform actions that don't align with your values or objectives.

The cognitive process of decision-making also plays a vital role in shaping our behavioral actions. If we perceive a situation in a positive light, we will take action to escalate the perception. This is also known as classical conditioning. It's how you transition from viewing that stylish red sports car to believing that you need it and must have one. The car becomes a representation of something else in your life that you would also like – whether that's freedom, status, or power.

This is where mind control tactics come into play. People use these strategies to shape human behavior in ways that benefit them and their objectives. By influencing how you perceive things in your environment, these tactics can bypass the rational mind. This is why it's easy to see why there are many misconceptions about how mind control and brainwashing work.

The Dangers of Mind Control

There is a fine line between manipulating human behavior and causing psychological trauma on an individual. People who use mind control techniques are usually aware of this and know their limits. However, others who use unethical practices to shape others' behavior can cause serious long-term effects (such as personality disturbances or destruction).

Mind control and brainwashing tactics can backfire because they can be used against the user. In fact, this is what caused the downfall of many historical cults throughout time. When the leader or guru of a group decides to use these tactics to oppress followers, they will often turn violent to defend themselves. When this happens, people who have been manipulated often go on a rampage against their former abusers and captors.

Suggestion

Suggestion is a form of mind control in which ideas are presented to an individual without their conscious awareness. One of the oldest forms of suggestion comes from hypnosis. This is a highly controversial practice that dates back to ancient times. It involves placing someone into a trance state and suggesting behaviors or ideas that can potentially cause long-term changes in their behavior.

The power of suggestion plays an important role in our everyday lives, whether or not we realize it. Many self-help books and public speakers use this strategy to get people to change their behaviors. For example, if you're a smoker who wants to quit, chances are you will be bombarded with suggestions from friends and family members on how you should quit. They may even present suggestions in the form of a plan that will help them quit smoking.

They are used to help people overcome addictions by giving them the support and motivation they need to change their behaviors. Many books detail how to quit smoking as well.

Yet, when these strategies are used against non-smokers, it can be called "mind control" or "brainwashing." Nevertheless, if you understand how suggestion works and how it forms the foundation of most mind control techniques, it becomes easier to see why this occurs.

The power of suggestion is also used in advertising to shape consumer behavior. The media gave us messages that are carefully crafted to make us feel a certain way. If you take the time to analyze ads, you will see that they are designed to make a particular product seem appealing. Whether it's an automobile, restaurant, or luxury item, the ad is designed to get you pre-programmed for a certain response.

In most cases, this is done through classical conditioning. It is a form of learning that occurs due to association. For example, if you used to eat at a certain restaurant because it smells good, has delicious food, and the service is always great, over time, you will develop positive associations with the place. Eventually, the thought of eating at that restaurant alone will make you feel good.

The same thing applies when you watch a particular TV commercial for a certain product. By repeating exposure to ads over time (along with other factors), you can eventually develop positive feelings towards them.

Notes

Chapter 8:
Mind Control in Popular Culture versus Mind Control in Reality

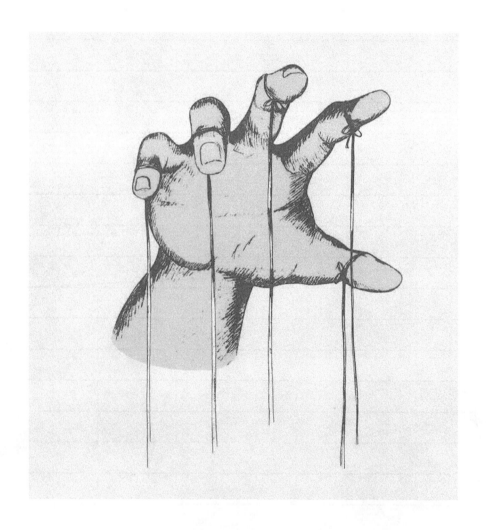

I n popular culture and the media, mind control has been a favorite topic of discussion. Mind Control is practiced by cult
leaders, psychiatrists, and the government. But, in reality, it is not
used that often for several reasons. Firstly, a person cannot be
made to do something against his will because his mind or consciousness will resist the influence of mind control. Secondly, it
takes years of training to perfect the techniques and, as such, requires a highly skilled practitioner who has devoted his life to this
art. Lastly, mind control is not worth it as the person involved is
left with no self-esteem, dignity, or identity of his own.

Mind Control in Reality versus Mind Control in Popular Culture

The mind-control techniques that exist in reality are not those
that are shown in popular culture. Some of the mind-control techniques mentioned in popular culture include hypnosis, electro-
convulsive therapy, drugs, and even inserting microchips into the
brain. In reality, most of these have been proven ineffective when
it comes to changing personalities and controlling minds.

A technique used by cults is called thought-stopping. Thought-
stopping is a technique that blocks out any thoughts that are contrary to the cult's doctrine. This technique works if the person has
to have some self-awareness of their own thoughts and desires. It
is only through this recognition that they can block out certain
thoughts and desires from their mind. This is why people who are

more intelligent and have a stronger personality and character are more resistant to this technique. Thought-stopping also gives the individual the feeling that his own thoughts are wrong.

However, a technique that is more effective in controlling and changing the personality is reality-stopping. Reality-stopping uses several mind control techniques and can be customized to fit the needs of the cult leader. Reality-stopping blocks out all outside influences from the individual's environment so that they are left with only one point of view, which is that of their leader. Any type of questioning or doubt that may exist on their part will be overridden by their cult leader, and he will start believing in what he is being told. This creates a cult of personality around the leader, and it is this technique that results in some of the atrocities that have occurred, such as mass killings, suicides, and sexual abuse.

The main principles of reality-stopping include:

1. Control of the Physical Environment: The physical environment in which the individual exists will be controlled by their leader to align with their wishes and desires. For example, controlling what type of media they are exposed to or what books and magazines they read will influence their thoughts and hence, their personality.

2. Control of Information: This is a technique that leaves the individual with only one point of view or perspective on certain issues. By having access to only one point of view, the individual does not have a choice, and they are instructed what to believe in and how to behave.

3. Thought-Stopping: This is a technique used by cults to stop certain thoughts from developing into beliefs contrary to their doctrine. The individual is told to stop thinking certain thoughts as they will cause them to sin. Thoughts are regarded to be evil in this technique.

4. Reality Revision: As the name implies, reality revision is a way of changing your reality by modifying it to fit into someone else's wishes and desires. In this technique, the person is told that certain thoughts and feelings are wrong. This leads to a contradiction in their mind such that they do not know what to think or feel. This is a technique used by cults to control and change their members' personalities and beliefs.

5. Guilt: The main aim of guilt is to make an individual believe that something he did was wrong or sinful. The individual will then become more eager to please the leader because he will think that he has sinned and needs forgiveness. Guilt is a powerful technique used by cults to keep their members in check.

6. Fear: Since the aim of the mind controller is to instill fear in his followers, they use various techniques to do so. The person may be told that if they leave the group, they will go to hell or

be punished for their beliefs and actions. They are also taught that if they disobey the cult leader, he will punish them severely.

How to Detect and Avoid Mind Control

If you are being controlled or manipulated, most likely, you don't even know about it. You may be so accustomed to the manipulative tactics that they appear "normal" to you. With that in mind, these are several things to watch out for:

Look for a slow erosion of your values and opinions. As time goes by, you notice that your opinions and beliefs keep changing (and changing back), depending on who is talking to you at the moment. This is a sign of having your core values reprogrammed by someone else's suggestions. You find yourself doing things you never saw yourself doing, such as lying to people you care about and other things that are just plain not like you. You find yourself buying things that don't make sense for your life but somehow seem attractive at the time. This is a sign of being influenced by other people's desires and motivations. You feel like someone else is "pulling the strings" of your life.

Look for sudden changes in your emotions. Your emotions change for no apparent reason, or they change in a pattern that you have never experienced before. Your inability to control your emotions keeps you from acting the way that feels right to you. You find yourself attracted to other people who have no interest in you and repulsed by those who do. This is a sign that some person or influence is causing very strong feelings — whether positive or negative — that you cannot control on your own. You feel like an outsider in your own life. Expressing your feelings, interests, and opinions makes you feel like a stranger to yourself.

How to avoid mind control

Don't be in a hurry to make decisions. When you have to make a difficult choice, don't rush into it. Take some time and analyze the options carefully. Don't let yourself be manipulated into making choices by someone else's opinions or emotions. Make your own decision by gathering all the facts you can get and then carefully thinking things through from all angles — inside and out. Don't be afraid to change your mind. You are free to change your mind at any time. In fact, you should always be ready to change your mind if the facts warrant it. Just make sure that you have all the facts available before making a decision.

Don't be afraid to say "no." If you don't feel right about doing something (for example, going along with someone else's manipulations or controlling ideas), then simply say no. It's that simple. If you feel that others are trying to control you, politely tell them that you will follow your own path and do your own thing for now. They can change their behavior, or they can leave you alone. The choice is theirs.

Ways to protect yourself from Mind Control techniques:

- Protect yourself from unethical "Psycho-Babble" sales pitches. Don't let anyone make you feel bad for being a skeptic. Trust your own instincts; they are smarter than you think they are. Using your critical thinking skills to differentiate between reality and the hype.

- Avoid being around negative or manipulative people who try to convince you that their way is the right way and that anyone who thinks differently is wrong.

- Don't let yourself be intimidated into doing something that feels wrong. If people pressure you in any way, turn to someone else for help if necessary. Don't be afraid or embarrassed to admit that you need help.

- Don't let yourself be pressured to make a decision until you have all of the necessary facts in front of you. Be your own judge and jury and make your own decisions based on what feels right inside of you.

- Don't be afraid to ask questions, say "I don't know," or admit when you are wrong. You don't have to have all of the answers, nor do you have to pretend that you do. Remember, your primary responsibility is to be true to yourself.

- Don't be afraid to take your time and think things through. If you have the tendency to make snap decisions, learn how to rewire your brain. Make a promise to yourself not to make any major decisions for at least twenty-four hours after you first hear about it. Give yourself a chance to absorb all of the information and think things through.

Notes

Chapter 9:
How to Use Mind Control

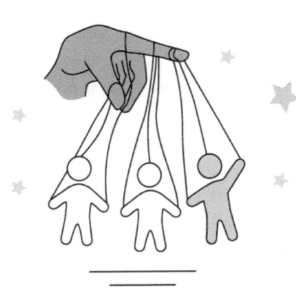

M ind control is a hot topic nowadays. Movies and TV shows are currently in love with the idea of mind control, and some have been accused of exposing people to subliminal messages while bewitching their audiences. Mind control, or more specifically, subliminal messaging, is a hot topic, but most people have no idea what it truly means and how powerful the results can be when you understand how their minds work.

According to scientists, your brain does everything it can to optimize processing power. It can do this by using one of two methods. It will reuse information it has already processed before or take shortcuts and make assumptions. A common example of the use of shortcuts in the brain can be seen if you hear a song playing on the radio. Even if you have not heard that song in years, your brain may begin singing along. This is because it takes shortcuts based on what has been previously learned and assumes something is familiar even if your conscious mind does not "recognize" the melody as anything important. The more you are exposed to something and ingrained it in your memory, it becomes a part of your life.

This is one of the most basic concepts of mind control. You have to give your target (the person you are trying to influence) a reason to make a subconscious connection. If your target can be exposed to something repeatedly by a trusted source, they will begin making assumptions and taking shortcuts in their brain.

Mind control can be used to reinforce positive habits or break unwanted ones. A good example of this is using it to reinforce a daily fitness regimen. Your target will not remember consciously that they should work out each morning. They may have forgotten about the last time they went to the gym, but their brain will remember that it felt good when they did work out and make replicating that feeling its priority. You can use this to break unwanted habits as well. For instance, a person that may be addicted to hard drugs could be exposed to something like a picture of a person suffering from addiction and overdose every day until they eventually feel uncomfortable whenever they feel the urge to get high. This is about using psychology and mind control on your target. They may not know what is influencing them, but your target most likely will not be happy with the results.

Being exposed to subliminal messaging daily will have a psychological impact on your target. You need to understand that it can be used for good or evil and adjust your message accordingly.

If you want to break a habit that someone has had for years, you must be patient. You cannot expect to expose them to your message daily and have it work the first time. It is a process you must consistently tap into daily on a subconscious level.

You need to be careful about what message you use, though, because this can either enhance the negative effects of their bad habit or reverse it completely. It is best to use something like a picture, a part of something, or even an idea. It doesn't need to elaborate, but it should be something you believe will resonate with your target. You can create your own message to send out subliminally.

Every week you should start seeing some effects, and then every month you will notice even more. Then after 3 months, you could have a completely different person on your hands. Rewiring someone's brain takes time; you must be consistent, but it will happen, and if you are relentless about it, you can even use it to create miracles.

A powerful example of this would be a person that is afraid of drowning. If you were exposed to water every day but never actually got wet, it would not take long for you to become desensitized to it. This is basically what you are doing to your target when you expose them daily for hours at a time with your message. They may not even remember why they felt so strongly about the thing in the first place because their brain will not allow them access to those memories and simply rewire itself instead.

This is scary stuff if you really think about it, but you can use subliminal messages to your advantage, and if you are patient and persistent, you can rewire someone's mind to do just about anything.

Notes

Chapter 10:
Empathy and Dark Psychology

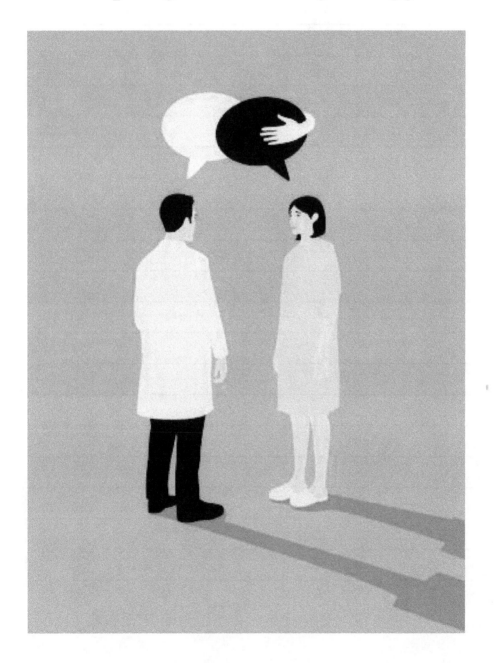

E mpathy is described as the ability to be sensitive and re-
sponsive to others' needs, whereas Dark Psychology is defined as an attempt to understand criminals' mindset.

Despite being opposites, empathy and dark psychology are two
concepts that overlap. The choice for people to engage in dark
psychology is ultimately up to them, but those with high levels of
empathy will be less likely to do so. Although rare, there are cases
where empathetic individuals have engaged in dark psychological
acts such as murder.

The different situations that arise within the context of dark psychology and empathetic disposition have been documented in
history. One such case is that of Albert Fish, who tortured and
killed at least fifteen children in New York in 1918. Fish was a pe-
dophile who not only killed his victims but also mutilated their
bodies. After being caught and sentenced to death, Fish expressed
no regret for his acts. He even wrote to the judge while awaiting
his death: "I still make my death mask. I am not afraid to die."
The quote highlights Fish's lack of empathy. In fact, Fish had a
history of sadistic abuse against children going back to 1900 when
he was only ten years old. Fish was an example of someone with
high levels of empathy who nonetheless had no remorse for his
actions.

There are also examples of empathetic people engaging in dark
psychological acts such as murder and torture. The Gestapo (Nazi
Secret Police) was an example. Although the Gestapo consisted of

men trained to torture, they were able to subject many people to unimaginable pain and terror. However, the act of torturing another person showed evidence of empathy within this group; it was a sign that the interrogators felt for their victims. It is possible that this empathy made their acts worse than if they had no emotional connection with their victims.

Even though some people have a natural disposition for empathy, they can still be prone to engaging in dark psychological acts depending on their circumstances. The circumstances involved in the choices to engage in these acts are related to family background and child-rearing techniques, among other things. Research indicates that abuse of children by their caregivers at an early age can cause them to develop antisocial, violent, or psychopathic tendencies.

A famous example is serial killer Ted Bundy, who was abused by his mother as a child. A boy who was abused may become an adult with low self-esteem and have a sense of inadequacy. He may then have to prove himself by engaging in dark psychological acts.

In the end, empathy plays an integral part in the choices that people make. Those who are empathetic will not engage in dark psychological acts, whereas those who feel little or no empathy are likely to do so.

A scale has been developed that attempts to measure a person's empathy levels based on their responses in certain situations and after answering a questionnaire. The three main components of empathy are affective, cognitive, and conative. The affective component is referred to as caring, whereas the cognitive component refers to being able to understand others' perspectives. The conative aspect is the ability to act on what you know about others and their needs. People who score high in empathy are better able to understand the feelings of those around them and act appropriately.

Dark Psychology is an important aspect of the scientific community. Psychologists attempt to understand what caused a person to commit a crime to avoid the recurrence of similar cases in the future. The overall goal of Dark Psychology is to be able to predict potential criminals and save civilians from being harmed by dangerous people.

Empathy and the Empath

Empathy is to be able to recognize and share the feelings of someone else. For you to do this, you must have the ability to see beyond yourself. Empathy does not mean that you are weak or spineless; it means that you can feel what others feel and care about it. For this reason, some people are unable to empathize with others because they are unable or unwilling to see beyond themselves. People like this usually put themselves at the center of their own little world and become narcissistic and selfish.

Empaths are quite the opposite of narcissists. Empaths are people who get what it is like to be someone else. They can sense the feelings of others, and they often develop a strong desire to help others. Most people are either empaths or narcissists, but some people have both empathic and narcissistic qualities.

One of the most important differences between empaths and narcissists is that empaths never take their eyes off other people. Empaths need to be able to see what other people see to understand how they feel. These people are very aware of themselves, but they are also very aware of everyone around them. This is why empaths do not crumble when they get negative feedback. Instead, they use the information to help them improve their relationships with others. Narcissists cannot take negative feedback because it makes them feel bad about themselves.

Empaths do not necessarily possess a high level of self-esteem. They simply have a better understanding of how other people think and feel. They are not the kind of people who view the world from their own point of view and think that is how everyone else should see it. Empaths know that everyone sees things differently, and they want to understand why. They do not judge people for their differences, and they strive to embrace these differences instead.

The Empath's Need for Control

Although empaths need to understand others' lives to make sense of their own, they are often unable to control their desire to help others. This is because they need to know what other people are feeling in order to understand for themselves. If a person feels confused or lost, an empath may feel this as if it were happening to them as well. Therefore, empaths have a tendency to try and control the feelings of people around them. They want to help these people, so they may try to take things into their own hands and fix the situation.

Empaths can become very controlling when they feel confused or lost themselves. They may become jealous of others or overly involved in their lives. Some empaths will even go so far as to tell other people how they should be feeling.

Empaths are not necessarily narcissistic or controlling, but they do struggle with other people's feelings. For this reason, empaths need to be able to recognize their own emotions in order to control them.

Notes

Chapter 11:
How to Use Empathy and then Get What You Want

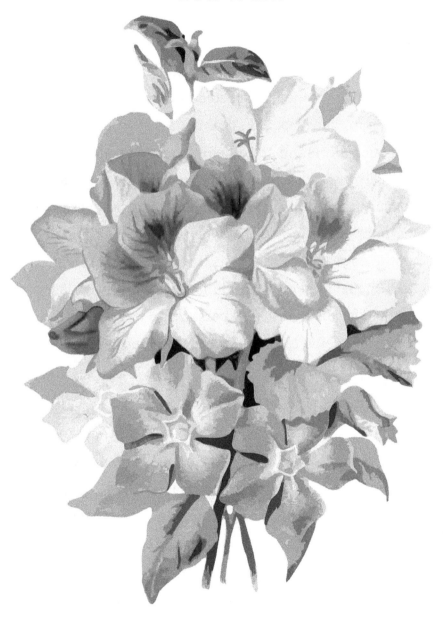

E mpathy is a tool used by many people to get what they want. Most people use empathy to help others without regard to their own self-interests. The first kind of empathy is often known as an empathic concern. This is the most basic aspect, and all forms of empathy follow this original aspect. Empathic concern is the ability for a person to understand that someone else is experiencing pain or suffering in some manner and then take action to stop or reduce that pain. It is a form of sympathy because the person not only knows the other is hurting but also feels some kind of negative emotion for the other person and that they want to do something about it. This can be illustrated by an example of two dogs fighting in the street. A person driving by can easily notice that the dogs are hurting each other. They don't need to stop and check on them; they just know that something bad is happening, and they feel bad for it. The person also has an idea of what could be done to stop the dogs from hurting each other. This is called empathic concern.

The next level of empathy that many people are familiar with is called compassionate empathy. This is where you empathize with someone, but you take it a step further and want to help that person. It's important to make them feel better or stop their suffering, so you will do what it takes to help them feel better or stop suffering. This kind of empathy can be thought of in the same terms as helping a friend through a hard time emotionally or maybe taking care of an injured animal. You don't want them to hurt, so you will do what you can to make them feel better. This is often described as "sinking into" another person's shoes. You try to imagine how you would feel if you were them and then do whatever it takes to help them. Many people often feel that they have to help those in need of such empathy.

The last type of empathy is often called perspective-taking empathic concern. This is the most advanced form of empathy that takes empathic concern and adds the aspect of attempting to see it from another's perspective to understand why they are suffering or hurting so much. This type of empathy leads someone to want to understand a foreign culture better or get in another person's mindset. The goal here is to stop the suffering, but you have to understand the other person in order to do it. Any time you try to understand another person or culture, you are using this kind of empathy. This is the type of empathy that leads to tolerance and understanding.

This type of empathy will be essential to get what you want and achieve your goals. Imagine on a moment that you are on a job interview or trying to persuade someone into doing something for you. You can't just ask for the things you want; you have to make them want to give it to you as well. The most successful approach is to try to understand what would make them want to provide you with what you want. Think of this as an explanation of why you want something.

The mistake most people make is just trying to tell people why they should help them or do what they want, and this doesn't work. It is no different from the dogs fighting in the street; people just see that you want something, and they don't care. If you want them to care, you have to show them how it is in their best interest to help you. This means that you have to show them how helping you will make their life better or easier. You are making an emotional argument instead of a logical one, and all good arguments need emotion.

The key here is trying to understand what would make someone want something and then give it to them. It works the same way for the job interview as it does for getting your kids to eat their dinner. Empathy can make people want to help you or help them feel better, but they have to comprehend that it is in their best interest. If you try to demand that people do what you want, it won't work; empathy must come first before any good argument can be made.

The Dark Psychology Worldview Compared to Empathetic Worldview

It is very obvious that almost any problem in society is a consequence of the predominantly empathetic worldview. This view holds that we are all "people," and we are all fundamentally identical. Thus, when someone does bad things to others, they must be doing bad things to themselves (or have been conditioned into doing these actions). The dark psychological worldview is the antithesis of these ideas.

The Dark Psychological Worldview

At the center of the dark psychological worldview is an understanding of how human beings actually work. The dark psychological viewpoint accepts that we are not all "people," nor are we all fundamentally identical. In fact, we are animals with extremely competitive urges as well as the urge to cooperate with others for mutual benefit. We have instincts to kill, rape, and steal from each other and instincts to nurture and help others (including strangers). We are born with these instincts, and we have evolved as a species over thousands of years.

Empathetic Worldviews in Action

The empathy-based solutions to our problems work like this: if someone is hurtful toward others, it is because they have been hurt by others. They must have a reason for their behavior. And if they do not have a reason, then we must "reason" with them and tell them to be nice to others. We will give them love and understanding. We will offer them rehabilitation opportunities through which they can learn better behaviors from the friendly, helpful people around them. We will forgive their past transgressions and give them another chance to do the right things (this is why we let repeat offenders out of prison). Even if all of the above fails, we will lock them up in comfortable prisons and hope that they reform in their golden years.

If such extreme measures fail, then there is no other option but to execute or imprison these "bad people." Most empathetic people would rather see suffering inflicted on themselves or their loved ones than see someone suffer who has done bad things.

Another empathetic worldview is based on the idea that people (who are fundamentally equal) do not cause problems; society causes problems. If there are problems in society, then it must be because we have not implemented enough empathy-based approaches to solving human nature. We will reform society by offering love and understanding to those who hurt others. We will strive to rehabilitate those who hurt others, and we will forgive their past transgressions. This is why we have so many "prison reformation" measures in society today and other social programs designed to help people (even those who do not want help). We live here in a society that does not let people die on the streets or starve to death. It does this because it is an empathetic society that wants to fix the problems of human nature. This is the society that we all have in common.

Humans Are Very Different – We Are Not All "People"

What if there really are problems with human nature? What if the empathy-based solutions are not fixing these problems? Then it is time to ask why there are problems with human nature in the first place. If the empathetic worldview is correct, then people do not cause problems. Rather, society causes problems because it has not provided enough welfare, housing programs, job training programs, etc.

It is very essential to understand that the vast majority of people who are hurtful toward others do not have a well-thought-out plan to be hurtful. They act out the urges within them when they are not stopped or punished. This is a very important thing for us to understand because it means that most people in society are not "bad." If we take this idea to its logical conclusion, we will realize that most people in society would never hurt others if they were left alone. But they are not left alone. Often they are kept on the streets because of their own "bad behaviors" when they would otherwise be able to contribute positively.

At this moment, the empathetic worldview may fail you. It tells us that people are fundamentally equal ("people") and that we all hurt each other. Unless there is a "reason" for someone's bad behavior, then there is no reason to lock them up or lock them out of society (we will just ignore them).

Notes

Chapter 12:
Dark Psychology and You

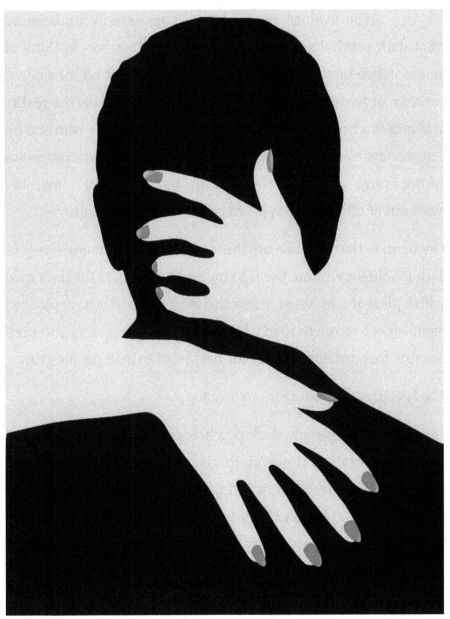

W hat you don't know about dark psychology can hurt you.

The average person doesn't necessarily understand what dark psychology is or how it works. Most people think of manipulative tactics as being anything that might be considered negative or harmful in any manner. While this is true, the reality of things is a little bit different. You see, most people who end up being categorized under the umbrella of having a 'dark psychology' are doing so because they are maybe looking for something more out of life than what is offered to them by default.

The truth is that just like anything else, there are many levels to dark psychology. Some use it to try and hurt others for their own selfish pleasure; however, there also exist those who have pledged themselves to a rough road where their purpose is simply to keep pushing forward and looking for new ways to help people grow.

The Realities of What Dark Psychology

For any normal person, dark psychology is generally considered something negative. However, this is because to the fact that most people are not interested in taking the time to really understand what it really is. Instead, they judge it by what they know of mental manipulation or what they see on television or movies.

So if you decided that you wanted to explore some of these things and see if there is a side of life that still has more to offer than what your life currently presents you with, where do you start?

The truth is that there are no real guidelines for beginning. You can read about dark psychology, and you can listen to what other people have to say about it. However, what you will find is that if you really want to understand it and use it effectively, you're going to need to begin on your own.

Dark psychology isn't generally believed to be something that people can use to abuse others. However, this is not the case. As with anything else in life, there will always be those who choose to take the path of least resistance and do whatever it takes to get what they want.

While I've said that most people begin their exploration into dark psychology out of a desire for something better than what their current situation holds for them, others don't quite see it this way. They maybe have been hurt in some way, or they might just not see the light at the end of their tunnel. These individuals are either trying to exact revenge upon someone who has hurt them in some way, or they are simply so lost that they don't know what else to do.

Once you begin your journey down this road, you must take the time to really think about what it is you want out of it. Remember, there are no real guidelines for how dark psychology should be used. I believe that a firm rule of thumb for anyone wanting to really dig into this area would be that the best thing you can do is use it for your own growth and never allow it to be used to hurt those around you.

If you can do this, you will not only have a clear conscience, you will also discover that once you begin using it in this manner, the benefits are far-reaching.

As you explore these concepts and ideas more and more, I am certain that you will find yourself going through many different levels of understanding. Don't be surprised if it takes some time to wrap your mind around everything connected to dark psychology. This is because it is an extremely rich area of study and one that can easily take up each moment of your time if you allow it to do so.

As a beginning student in this area, you should not be surprised if this is exactly what happens. The reason for this saying is because the only person who can really get to the bottom of these things is you.

Chapter 13:
10 Ways to Become a Super-Likable Person using Dark Psychology

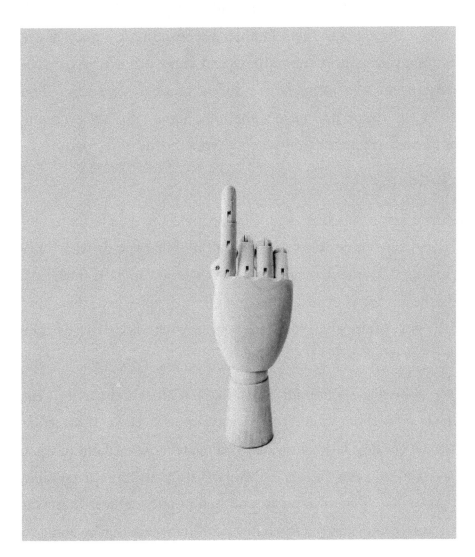

A lot of my writing so far has been on how to become a bad person, but now it's time to turn that around and think of ways you can become the most likable person around. I've collected ten ways to do it, and they're incredibly powerful. Some of them might seem familiar because they're tips that are always given to us. None of these will make you a 'nice guy' because niceness is boring. If you follow these strategies you'll be fun to be around and have something about you that everyone wants more of. Be that guy who's always the life of the party.

1. Be Funny

No, not just make jokes and have people think you're funny. Be audaciously funny. Jokes are fine, but it's what you do with them that count. Think about making people laugh so hard they can't breathe anymore, or just smile and give a giggle when something really isn't funny at all. You can be funny with body language or even just how you act in general.

Keep your sense of humor sharp like a scalpel and use it to cut people up without them becoming aware of it. How? If someone insults you, take it dead serious and make a big deal out of what they said. You can do this by bringing it up at the next possible opportunity, which will be around in a minute or two. Then you can 'laugh' it off and put them in a position where they're going to seem like they've made a terrible mistake. They'll learn to be more careful around you if you can do this properly. It's all about biting people behind their backs while they don't even know it, and that's what makes people likable.

2. Be the Life of the Party

As I said before, niceness is boring. Boring people get no love. You have to be the guy who's always cracking jokes, who's always the center of attention, and who gets everyone laughing all the time. Be that man or woman everyone looks forward to seeing at parties. If someone's hosting and you're the guest of honor, get people laughing left, right, and center about everything going on that day.

If you can do this well enough, people will want to know your secrets, and they'll like to hang out with you 24/7. Whatever you do, don't give it up because it will be worth your while later on. This is the kind of person that everyone wants as a friend because they make everyone else feel like they're at the top of their game themselves. Respect comes from likability, so this is how you earn it in no time flat.

3. Compliment, Compliment, Compliment

Everyone loves a compliment, so why not give it out like candy? But don't just stick to the normal compliments that everyone else tells you. You want to compliment when people least expect it because that's what makes you stand out. Make it really odd too, like saying something about a person's shoelaces and how they go perfectly with their shirt. If you're creative and can see what others aren't noticing, you're on the right track to becoming more likable.

Compliments can make people feel good about themselves, and that's what most of the population is looking for anyway. Everyone wants to be accepted, and compliments are the quickest way to let them know you like them. They'll be seeking you out for more, and they'll want to spend time with you more often if you're always giving out great compliments. That's how you become a likable person.

4. Give Other People Attention

If you're always giving people attention, they'll want to give you attention right back. You should be acting like total royalty when it comes to compliments and not treating them like they are nothing special at all. If you can do this to each person who gives you a compliment, then they'll remember it forever.

Make sure people know what you've done too. Tell them your accomplishments every time you get a chance. People love to hear things like that because it makes them feel good about themselves as well. When they tell people about you, they'll be saying the same things you've been saying, and then you'll get more attention. That's how it works, so put yourself out there and give people some of your time.

5. Be Different

Everyone wants to fit in, but that's not the only way to become likable. Be different from everyone else and stand out as a result. This doesn't necessarily mean you're a weirdo; it just means you are your own person. People will come to admire that because everyone else is too scared to be themselves for fear of the consequences. You'll be going against the grain and making your presence known.

Don't be afraid to show you've got your own style by wearing whatever you want. If someone says something about it, thank them, like they complimented you on something nice. Be yourself no matter what, because if you try to be someone else, you'll just end up getting called out on it. If people like the real version of you, then why not give them that?

6. Be the Showy Type

If you really want to be more likable and get more attention, then be showy. This doesn't necessarily mean being an attention hog yourself, but it does mean not turning down an opportunity to get people's eyes on you. If there's a party, go in wearing the most outrageous-looking outfit you can find. People will be trying hard to know where you got it and how you pulled it off. If there's no party going on, then do something to make your presence known.

Show off and get people's attention by being completely okay with doing stupid things that no one else is willing to do in public. If you want to be more likable, then that's how you'll do it, and don't feel bad about it either.

If you do these things and treat them with respect, you'll make yourself a pretty likable person.

7. Don't Try So Hard When It Comes To Being Likable

Just a simple fact of life is that if you try too hard, then you'll end up looking desperate and uncool. If you're trying hard to be liked, then people will know it. This is why you have to act naturally when it comes to being likable. If you can do this, other people will believe you because they have the same reactions.

If you can act naturally when it comes to being likable, then other people will be able to respond in kind and like you back. If someone is acting in an unnatural way around you, then they're probably only trying to get something out of you. Don't let that person suck all the likability out of you; just walk away from them if it seems like they're up to something or not being themselves.

8. Don't Be Afraid To Put Yourself Out

If you're afraid to put yourself out and meet new people, then you might be putting off a vibe that you're not likable. Being likable means being willing to meet new people and make some friends. This isn't the same thing as being desperate, though.

If you don't want to have some kind of stigma attached to a personality trait of yours, then don't let fear dictate your life. You shouldn't be afraid to sit in the center of a room or go up to talk to someone stranger at a social event. This is the only way you're ever going to succeed when it comes to making friends and being likable.

9. Relate To People

Simply put, if you can relate well with other people, then they'll be able to accept you easier than someone who doesn't share much of anything in common with them. Having common ground with people is important when it comes to being likable. It also means that you won't have to strain your brain trying to find things to talk about with them.

10. Be a Good Listener

Having a conversation is easy but actually listening in on one is much harder. If you want people to really like you, you're going to have to learn how to listen and pay attention. Don't wait for your turn to talk or cut the other person off. A good listener also makes a good friend. If you don't feel like listening to someone, tell them you think you are tired and ask if they'll meet up again later.

A caring listener is a good friend. Caring Listener will easily get friends, respect, and higher social status. When you listen carefully to others' problems and concerns, they feel grateful and want to help you back.

Find ways to be genuinely interested in others and their lives, and they'll feel so good about sharing themselves with you. If you give advice without being asked for it and show genuine care for the person, they're going to see that you're a good person who can be trusted with anything.

Even if you don't have the time to help someone out and you can't be of much use to them, still offer your support. If they want advice, then give it but be sure that it comes from the heart and is really something that's meant to help them.

These Good traits in Dark Psychology may help you make friends and bring success in life.

Notes

Conclusion:

D ark Psychology is real. As discussed, the dark side of human nature is real too.

Reality is a constant battle between good and evil. Once you recognize this, you will understand that our world is not the best it can be and that there are huge flaws within the human race that need to be corrected.

The truth is it's just in front of you; it's just a matter of whether you are brave or crazy enough to accept it and face it.

Knowledge of Dark Psychology is important because it can help us open our eyes and appreciate what we have, make better decisions about life, understand other people's motivations better and most importantly, save our own lives and those of others.

It is better to know the truth than to be ignorant. Ignorance may be bliss, but it is also extremely dangerous. If you do not grasp the reality of our situation, you will not be prepared when things get tough. But if you do, you will be ready to face whatever is thrown at you with courage and wisdom.

What is the point of undergoing the best training and learning fighting skills if you don't even realize when you are about to get in a fight?

And let's not forget that Dark Psychology is not just limited to physical violence. It very much includes emotional violence, manipulation, and abuse. We must learn how to protect ourselves and our loved ones from these dark forces as well. We must know what kind of danger we are in to protect ourselves from it.

Sometimes, you may think that you must live in blissful ignorance to keep your life simple and stress-free. This way, you don't need to deal with any painful thoughts or uncertainties.

It is not easy to be aware and accept the fact that people are trying to "get one over" on us at all times, but this is how our world works. The truth is that you can also do it to others if you have the knowledge and skills.

Thank you for reading the book until the end; I hope you have learned something valuable from this book.

Notes